NATURAL TREATMENTS FOR

Urinary Incontinence

Using Butterbur and Other Natural Supplements to Treat Bladder-Control Problems

RITA ELKINS, M.H.

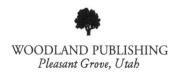

WOODLAND PUBLISHING
Pleasant Grove, Utah

Woodland Publishing
P.O. Box 160
Pleasant Grove, Utah
84062
Visit us at our web site: www.woodlandbooks.com
or call us toll-free: (800) 777-2665

The information in this book is for educational purposes only and is not recommended as a means of diagnosing or treating an illness. All matters concerning physical and mental health should be supervised by a health practitioner knowledgeable in treating that particular condition. Neither the publisher nor the author directly or indirectly dispenses medical advice, nor do they prescribe any remedies or assume any responsibility for those who choose to treat themselves.

ISBN 1-58054-085-6
Printed in the United States of America.

CONTENTS

Introduction

URINARY INCONTINENCE AFFECTS millions of Americans and is no discriminator of age. Although urinary incontinence is usually associated as a side effect of aging, incontinence is commonly seen in younger people, especially women. Urinary incontinence can be a troublesome, not to mention embarrassing, problem. Successfully treating incontinence depends on targeting the cause of the problem.

Several herbs have recently emerged that may have extraordinary therapeutic benefit for anyone with incontinence; a number of complementary compounds can help manage disorders of the bladder and urinary system. Combining natural medicine with Kegel exercises, biofeedback, acupuncture, and so forth makes for a much more effective therapeutic strategy.

This booklet is designed to provide a complete overview of both conventional and alternative medicine options for treating urinary incontinence. While several natural substances can help tone and cleanse the urinary tract, if your incontinence stems from a structural problem, you may need to go beyond the use of supplementation. Learning about urinary incontinence, the latest treatments and natural remedies will enable you to approach your health care practitioner with the knowledge and confidence you need to make educated decisions.

Urinary Incontinence: An Overview

Thankfully, open discussions about urinary incontinence are common today, a fact that will hearten anyone who has to deal with the problem. Conservative estimates tell us that one in ten seniors must cope with the condition; however, more realistic figures place that amount at over 30 percent. Urologists estimate that seventeen million Americans suffer from incontinence, and 85 percent of these sufferers are women. Approximately half of all women experience urinary incontinence at some time during their lives and suffer from the condition twice as often as men.

What does this mean in real numbers? As many as twenty-five million Americans cope with some degree of incontinence, and many of these people do not discuss the problem with their physicians. In fact, it is estimated that over half of all people with incontinence don't report it to their doctors. In many cases, incontinence develops as the urinary systems age and contributing diseases appear. Twenty percent of the elderly and 50 percent of nursing home residents have incontinence. In fact, urinary incontinence is one of the most common reasons elderly people are placed in nursing homes.

Some 40 percent of women over the age of sixty experience incontinence. Many relatively young women also suffer from some form of incontinence, and many of these women suffer in silence. Women are particularly prone to incontinence because pregnancy and childbirth can weaken the muscles that control urination.

Fortunately, several options are available for treating urinary incontinence, and in many cases, the condition may be reversible. Discovering the real cause of incontinence is crucial to selecting the most effective treatment. Understand that incontinence should not be viewed as an inevitable consequence of aging. If left untreated, incontinence can cause rashes and skin infections, not to mention depression, embarrassment, social withdrawal and anxiety.

DEFINITION OF URINARY INCONTINENCE

Urinary incontinence refers to the involuntary loss of urine. Most cases of incontinence are due to a weakening of the sphincter muscle that keeps urine in the bladder. The condition is also referred to as a bladder control problem, which can fall into one of three categories: an overactive bladder; sphincter muscle abnormalities (also called stress incontinence); and mixed incontinence, which involves a combination of both overactive bladder and sphincter malfunctions. Overactive bladder problems are very common and are not linked to normal aging processes that take place in the urinary system. People with an overactive bladder feel an urgent need to urinate frequently and may even leak urine. Overactive bladder disorder makes day-to-day living difficult in that you feel you can never be too far from a bathroom facility.

FIND OUT THE CAUSE OF URINARY INCONTINENCE

Urinary incontinence is a symptom of an underlying condition. Visiting your doctor or health practitioner and thoroughly describing your symptoms is an important first step to successful treatment. Without a complete medical exam, your doctor won't be able to determine why the problem exists. All kinds of treatments exist for incontinence, and it is commonly cured or, at the very least, managed well enough to permit an active lifestyle with little or no restriction. The worst thing you can do is nothing.

Left untreated, urinary incontinence can cause considerable physical and emotional damage. The longer incontinence is left untreated, the more susceptible you are to urinary tract infections, sores, rashes and so on. Equally important is the negative impact that incontinence has on self-esteem: depression and social withdrawal are commonly seen consequences of the condition.

Because the risk of an accident is always on the minds of people with incontinence, these individuals often avoid going out with friends or participating in any physical activity. However, a variety of treatment options are available; even if incontinence cannot be fully reversed, it can certainly be managed to the point where the quality of life is no longer compromised. Before we discuss incontinence in more detail, let's take a look at the workings of the urinary system.

Production, Storage and Release of Urine

At any given time, your kidneys are busy filtering impurities out of one-fourth of your blood supply. More than two million filter units in the kidneys work to separate toxic compounds, excess nutrients and water from the blood. The kidneys also maintain the delicate pH (acid/alkaline) values of the blood by balancing appropriate sodium and potassium levels, which are vital to proper cellular function. The kidneys also reabsorb 90 percent of the filtered materials for re-use, and the kidneys produce specific hormones that help to regulate blood pressure and other body functions. The kidneys recycle about forty-five gallons of blood every day and contain 2.4 million nephron filters, which are made up of fifty miles of tiny capillaries and tubules.

After the kidneys have separated out enough water to maintain proper blood levels, this water, which mixes with other biochemicals, becomes urine. Urine then flows down a small tube called the ureter to the bladder, which is nothing more than a muscular storage pouch. If urine remains in the bladder for too long, irritation can occur, and bacteria can cause infection. As the bladder fills, it creates the urge to urinate. Your brain then sends a signal to relax the urethral sphincter muscle opening that comes out of the bladder, this muscle begins to contract, and urine flows out of the body thorough the urethra. Incontinence can result if any part of this system malfunctions.

Types of Urinary Incontinence

STRESS INCONTINENCE

Stress incontinence (SUI) is the involuntary loss of urine during coughing, sneezing, laughing, lifting or other physical activities that increase pressure on the abdomen. You may have also found that you experience urine leakage when you rise from a sitting position, get out of bed, jog or do other exercises. SUI can occur when muscles that make up the pelvic floor lose their tone after childbirth, weight gain, certain surgeries, or with aging. Menopause or premenstrual conditions can worsen SUI because reduced levels of estrogen can aggravate the problem. SUI occurs when certain muscles stretch over time, causing the neck of the bladder to droop. This unnatural position causes the bladder neck to open when any pressure on the abdomen increases, such as when you sneeze or cough. SUI can also occur when the set of muscles responsible for squeezing the opening around the urethra becomes weak.

SUI has no link with emotional stress and is strictly a physical problem. People with SUI go to the bathroom several times a day to avoid leakage problems. SUI occurs primarily in women but can also develop in men, especially after prostate or other pelvic surgery. SUI is considered a common condition and can often be corrected.

URGE INCONTINENCE

Urge incontinence (UI) is an involuntary loss of urine that is linked with experiencing an overpowering desire to void. UI can occur with certain neurological disorders but also commonly appears with no associated abnormality. People with UI start to leak urine as soon as they feel a strong urge to go to the bathroom. Accidents can occur when bathroom facilities are not readily accessible or after drinking even a small amount of liquid. The sound or touch of running water can also initiate urine leakage. Nighttime bedwetting and going to the bathroom frequently are often seen in cases of UI.

UI typically occurs when the muscles that help keep the bladder closed experience spasms, and control is lost. UI is sometimes referred to as overactive or unstable bladder. Reflex incontinence is also used to describe UI if the condition occurs from overactive nerves found in the muscles that work the bladder. Possible causes of UI include bladder or vaginal infections, trauma, nerve damage, alcohol consumption or as a side effect of some prescription drugs.

UI is commonly seen in people with diabetes, Parkinson's disease, multiple sclerosis, dementia, cerebral palsy, stroke victims and menopausal women due to a decline in estrogen. Some people with UI sustain tension in the muscles surrounding the bladder and its opening; consequently, they become unable to sense signals that their bladder is full. By then, control is lost. Other people suffer from bladder contractions that occur without warning.

OVERFLOW INCONTINENCE

Overflow incontinence (OI) is the involuntary loss of urine associated with overdistension of the bladder (that is, when the bladder becomes enlarged or stretched out of shape). OI may cause a variety of symptoms such as frequent dribbling, UI or SUI. OI is the most common form of incontinence in men suffering from an enlarged prostate gland. With OI, the bladder stays consistently full, causing small amounts of urine to continually leak from it. People with OI feel that their bladder is never completely emptied. The problem occurs throughout the day and night, and when you get up to go to the bathroom because your bladder feels full, you only lose small amounts of dribbling urine.

OI occurs in people with diabetes and in men who have an enlarged prostate gland, which blocks the flow of urine. Other possible causes of OI include tumors and kidney stones. Unlike other forms of incontinence, OI is considered serious and mandates immediate medical attention. If left untreated, it can cause urine to flow back into the kidneys, which increases the risk of kidney infection and possible permanent damage. OI is rarely seen in women.

Note: SUI and UI are the two most common types of incontinence. About 70 percent of urinary incontinence cases are the UI type, characterized by uncontrollable bladder contractions that create the need to urinate and result in the leakage of urine.

FUNCTIONAL INCONTINENCE

Functional incontinence (FI) describes urine loss caused by conditions that exist outside the lower urinary tract and that impair normal function. FI has nothing to do with abnormal bladder function. It happens as a side effect of another seemingly unrelated condition such as Alzheimer's disease, in which case the person has lost the ability to plan to reach a toilet facility in time. Confinement to a wheelchair or other debilitating conditions can also cause FI.

TRANSIENT INCONTINENCE

Transient incontinence (TI) describes temporary bouts of incontinence. TI can result from the use of certain prescription drugs, the presence of urinary tract infections, mental illness, severe constipation or from being bedridden for a long period of time.

Summary of Symptoms of Incontinence

• leaking urine while exercise, laughing, coughing, sneezing or lifting
• consistent loss of dribbling urine

- inability to hold urine long enough to reach a bathroom facility
- urine smell on clothes and in the house.

Warning Signs of Bladder Problems

If you are experiencing any of the symptoms listed below, visit your doctor.

- urine leakage
- inability to urinate (retention of urine)
- urinating more frequently than usual without the presence of a bladder infection
- losing urine if you do not get to the bathroom fast enough
- pain or burning related to filling the bladder or emptying the bladder in the absence of a bladder infection
- frequent bladder infections
- progressive weakness of the urinary stream with or without incomplete bladder emptying
- abnormal urination or changes in urination related to stroke, spinal cord injury, multiple sclerosis, Alzheimer's disease and so on
- blood in the urine

Possible Causes of Incontinence

Urinary incontinence is not considered a natural part of aging. It can occur at any age and can be caused by many physical conditions. Incontinence is frequently just temporary and can be managed with simple treatment. Some causes of incontinence include the following:

- urinary tract infection
- vaginal infection or irritation
- constipation
- side effects of medicine or radiation therapy
- pelvic injury or surgery
- neurological diseases such as Parkinson's disease and multiple sclerosis
- strokes

- Alzheimer's disease
- prostatitis or benign prostate hypertrophy (BPH)
- diabetes
- cerebral palsy

When incontinence is due to structural problems, it will usually persist unless surgery, Kegel exercises and so forth are employed. In many cases, this condition can be treated after the cause has been determined. Some of the conditions that can cause incontinence due to structural problems include the following:

- childbirth
- a weakening of the muscles that hold the bladder in place
- a weakening of the bladder walls
- a weakening of the urethral sphincter muscles
- overactive bladder muscles
- a blocked urethra (such as from prostate enlargement)
- a lack of estrogen
- neurologic disorders
- immobility

What to Expect if You Go to Your Doctor

To get to the root of the problem, your doctor will usually take a medical history and perform a physical exam. A complete urinalysis is commonly done to rule out the presence of urinary infections. The following tests may also be administered:

- **Bladder capacity test:** This procedure determines how much urine your bladder holds when it is full. You drink an ample amount of water and then urinate into a container that measures volume.
- **Residual volume test:** This test determines how much urine actually stays in your bladder after you have urinated. A catheter is used to collect and measure any remaining urine.
- **Stress test:** This test is designed to pinpoint SUI. You will be asked to cough or strain your abdominal muscles while your doctor watches for any loss of urine.
- **Urodynamics:** These are tests that can measure the pressure

within your bladder and the rate at which urine flows out. These tests are usually administered by a urologist or urogynecologist.

• **Cystoscopy:** In this procedure, the doctor inserts a small tube through your urethra into your bladder to take a look inside.

• **Ultrasound:** This test give the doctor a view of your urinary tract from the outside. An ultrasound uses sound waves to create a visual image. A metal probe is moved across your skin to produce images of the kidneys, bladder, urethra and ureters.

Medical Treatments for Incontinence

Your treatment will depend on the type of urinary incontinence that you have. If an infection is present, it will be treated with prescription antibiotics. If an infection is ruled out, the most common types of medicines used are those that work to replace hormones, stop abnormal bladder muscle contractions or tighten sphincter muscles. These drugs include oxybutynin, propantheline and hyoscyamine. These medications also help to reduce the contractions that can cause UI. In addition, Detrol (tolteridine) may work for patients who have an overactive bladder or suffer from the frequent urge to urinate. Detrol works to block nerve impulses from the brain that signal the bladder to contract. Pseudoephedrine may also help strengthen a weak urinary sphincter muscle.

Hormone replacement therapy (HRT) may be recommended if incontinence seems directly related to a loss of estrogen. Imipramine, an antidepressant, has also been used in the past but is not currently prescribed as frequently due to its unwanted side effects. Another drug, desmopressin acetate, is an antidiuretic hormone sprayed in the nose that is sometimes tried but does not have a good history of long-term success. All of the above drugs have been associated with side effects that include headache, dizziness, dry mouth and blurred vision.

Non-Drug Therapies for Incontinence

KEGEL EXERCISES

Kegel exercises strengthen the pelvic and sphincter muscles of people suffering from SUI and can be quite effective. These exercises work to develop the pubococcygeous muscle, which contracts to stop urination. Kegel exercises can be especially valuable for women with SUI. You perform these exercises by deliberately stopping your urine flow two to three times. Even the elderly and those who have had incontinence for years can benefit from Kegel exercises.

To do Kegel exercises, you must first locate your pelvic floor muscles. The best way is to start urinating and then try to abruptly stop or slow the flow. If the amount of urine decreases, you are employing the right set of muscles. When you contract these muscles, you should feel a squeezing sensation around the urethra and the anus. Tighten this set of muscles for five seconds and then relax for five seconds. Begin by doing this exercise three to four times daily, and work up to holding each contraction for ten seconds several times a day. You can do this exercise in any position and at any time of the day.

Women also have the option of using vaginal weights to make the exercises even more effective. These weights are prescribed by your doctor and are inserted into the vagina. You must learn to squeeze the correct muscles to keep the weights from falling out.

The following will help you use Kegel exercises most effectively.

- Keep your stomach and buttock muscles relaxed.
- Don't hold your breath or clench any part of your body.
- Learn to contract the right muscles before sneezing or coughing.
- If you are not sure that you are doing these exercises correctly, consult your doctor.

Keep in mind that it may take several months to benefit from pelvic floor exercises, and doing them consistently is key. You can learn more about Kegel exercises online at http://www. mayohealth.org/mayo/9801/htm/incontirv.htm/pelvx.htm and http://my.webmd.com/content/dmk/dmk_article_5462622.

ELECTROSTIMULATION

This treatment supplements pelvic muscle exercises and strengthens muscles that help support bladder control. Electrostimulation can be used in people with SUI or UI. Electrical impulses are directed at the muscles involved to stimulate contractions.

MAGNETIC TREATMENT CHAIR

The Food and Drug Administration recently approved a new magnetic treatment designed to enhance pelvic floor muscle strength and support. This therapy is referred to as extracorporeal magnetic innervation and is only used for female patients with SUI, UI or mixed forms of incontinence. It is administered using a chair with built-in magnetic capabilities.

For this therapy, you are seated in the chair, and magnetic pulses are applied that cause contractions of the pelvic floor muscles and increase their strength. The magnetic pulses feel like a vibrating or tap-like sensation. You are not required to disrobe for the therapy. These treatments are administered in a doctor's office and typically last for less than thirty minutes. Sessions are repeated twice a week for two months. The effectiveness of this treatment has not yet been determined.

BLADDER TRAINING:

Learning to urinate on a set schedule, combined with biofeedback therapy, may help people with UI and OI. For people with FI, caregivers may also choose to use scheduled times for urination (prompted voiding). Bladder training can be effective for both men and women. Distraction, or thinking about other things, is another method for controlling UI.

BIOFEEDBACK THERAPY

In this therapy, electronic sensors are used to help the person understand what happens during bouts with incontinence so that control of the muscles involved in prior Kegel exercises can be used properly.

PESSARIES

This treatment is used for some cases of SUI in women. A pessary is a donut-shaped ring that is inserted into the vagina to help reposition the urethra.

IMPLANTS

In this treatment, a rubbery substance is injected around the urethra to help improve muscle control in people with SUI. Collagen injections are sometimes used for the same purpose. However, the success of this treatment is hard to predict.

URETHRAL PLUGS AND PATCHES

Small plugs can be inserted into the urethra and inflated to prevent urine leakage. A patch is a foam pad that sticks to the skin around the urethra to keep urine from leaking. These devices are sometimes effective in women suffering from mild incontinence.

SURGERY

When a physical obstruction is present that causes OI, surgery may be the only viable option. There are many different surgical procedures that may be used to treat incontinence. The type of operation you may need depends on the cause of your incontinence. In some cases of SUI, surgery may also be recommended if Kegel exercises and electrostimulation fail to strengthen the muscles supporting the bladder. Surgery can aid in the following ways:

- help restore the bladder neck to its proper position in women suffering from SUI
- remove tissue that may be causing an obstruction
- help strengthen weakened pelvic muscles
- expand the capacity of a small bladder to hold more urine

CATHETERIZATION

People with OI due to a structural obstruction who are not candidates for surgery may need to have a catheter inserted through the urethra to drain urine from time to time. Self-catheters are also available that help you completely empty your bladder.

PADS

Disposable pads and special underwear are commonly used with any of the above treatments.

Natural Therapies for Incontinence

As mentioned earlier, the success of any incontinence therapy depends on targeting the cause of the problem. The following sections describes possible dietary factors involved in certain types of incontinence and discusses herbs and other natural compounds that work to correct possible causes of incontinence. The secret to using natural medicines effectively is to be patient—natural treatments usually take longer to achieve desired results than do strong, potentially dangerous synthetic drugs. Moreover, for best results, also use Kegel exercises, biofeedback or other supplemental therapies.

Before you purchase any herbal medicine or natural compound, here are some guidelines to keep in mind:

- Purchase herbs and other natural compounds from reliable sources that you know are pure and have the desired potency. Look for standardized products with guaranteed potency.
- Take dosages that are recommended, and don't assume taking more is always better.
- If you are prone to allergies, pregnant, nursing or taking other drugs for any condition, check with your doctor before using herbs.
- Herbs are designed to work with the body and usually require consistent use over a long period of time to achieve the desired results.
- Try to use products from companies that are sympathetic to the environment and to ecological awareness.
- Read the product label for possible contraindications of herbs, and make sure you do not have a condition or are taking drugs that may cause an unwanted interaction.
- Keep all herbs and natural medicines, including vitamins and minerals, out of the reach of children.

Dietary Guidelines for Incontinence

For some people, especially children, milk allergies may play a part in certain cases of incontinence. A lactose intolerance should be ruled out. Avoid dairy products and substitute nondairy beverages, and keep a record of episodes of incontinence to establish a possible link to your diet. Try eliminating coffee and other forms of caffeine, tobacco and alcohol. Caffeine is found in milk chocolate, soft drinks and over-the-counter medications and is used in many baked goods and processed foods (although you won't find it listed on the labels). Drink pure water in reasonable amounts, and eliminate carbonated and other acidic beverages.

Coffee, milk, sugar, corn syrup, honey, alcoholic beverages, tea, soft drinks, chocolate, fruits, citrus juices, tomatoes or tomato-based products and spicy foods have been linked to some cases of incontinence. Keep a food diary to see if any correlation exists between what you consume and your incontinence.

Drink carrot, parsley, celery, cucumber, unsweetened black cherry and cranberry juices. Avoid high-fat, high-sugar diets that are heavy in refined flours. Increase your consumption of fresh, raw fruits and vegetables and whole grains, and avoid dairy products and artificial sweeteners. Watermelon seed tea and asparagus are also recommended for any malfunctions of the urinary system. If you think your incontinence may be related to constipation or bowel impaction, increase your consumption of whole, unprocessed, coarse wheat bran. Start using bran in small amounts, such as one tablespoon, and gradually increase the amount over time. Eating stewed prunes or using prune juice daily in combination with a magnesium supplement can also work wonders.

Herbs and Other Natural Compounds for Incontinence

The natural approaches to treating incontinence have been divided into treatment strategies based on the underlying cause of the condition. For example, if recurring bladder infections are a contributing factor to your incontinence, the condition should be treated with the appropriate herbs, such as cranberry, goldenseal and echinacea. If you are suffering from incontinence that is caused by the presence of prostate disease, using herbs that shrink the prostate gland can help to restore normal urinary function. Remember that herbs and other natural therapeutic agents work best when combined with Kegel exercises, biofeedback and other treatments. In general, the most effective herbal protocol would be to first try urinary system tonics that work to strengthen the urinary tract, and then work from there. You may have to experiment a little to arrive at your best treatment protocol.

The advantage of using natural compounds for incontinence is that unlike harsh drugs or drastic surgical procedures, alternative remedies are usually safe and come with little or no side effects. Use plant extracts and other compounds that work to build kidney and bladder tone, fight any possible infections and boost the overall workings of the urinary system when treating incontinence. The following compounds can be used to treat the urinary system.

HERBS FOR INCONTINENCE CAUSED BY MUSCLE SPASMS OF THE URINARY TRACT AND BLADDER

Butterbur *(Petasites vulgaris)* DESF or *(Petasites hybridus)*: Butterbur is a plant related to coltsfoot and grows in low-lying, marshy meadows and by riversides. Called *plague root* in Germany, it was used to treat plagues during the middle ages. It is considered a natural analgesic (pain reliever) and is generally nontoxic and nonaddictive. It is available in tablet form under the brand name of Petadolor in Germany and has recently emerged under other product labels in the United States.

Currently, renewed medical interest in butterbur has occurred because of its remarkable spasmo-analgesic effects. The spasmolytic activity of butterbur is primarily due to its primary active principle, a compound called petasin. This compound has cramp-relieving effects that some experts believe are fourteen times stronger than those of the muscle relaxant compound called papaverin. Experimental studies also show that petasin has pain relieving and sedating properties.

Butterbur root extract works to regulate and relax the bladder spasms that can create involuntary urination in certain cases. Some members of the German Commission E (a board that evaluates the therapeutic value and safety of herbal medicines) stand behind the ability of butterbur to successfully treat urinary tract colic.

One clinical trial using the herb involved two groups of twenty patients who were given one to two capsules of either a butterbur root preparation or butylscopolamin (a prescription drug) five times daily. Each group showed similar results: sixteen out of twenty patients in the group treated with butterbur root and eighteen out of twenty patients in the butylscopolamin group were free of pain from urinary tract spasms within twenty-four hours. Unlike butylscopolamin, however, the butterbur produced no side effects. In another study, butterbur was effectively used to treat an irritable bladder. The success of this application was supported by test results which showed that those who took butterbur root increased the length of time between urination from the third week of therapy onward. It is important to note that the effectiveness of butterbur is significant after four weeks of treatment and becomes even more pronounced after eight weeks.

Recommended Dosage: Tincture of butterbur extract can be used by taking a single drop in half a glass of water several times daily for a week; increase the dose to two drops the second week and then to three drops the next week. Butterbur extract tablets, called Petadolor, that dissolve on the tongue are currently available. Butterbur is now also available in capsules and should be taken according to label instructions.

Possible Side Effects: Butterbur root belongs to those plants containing natural sources of pyrrolizidinalkaloids. The German Health Department, Bundesgesundheitsamt (BGA), regulated pyrrolizidinalkaloids in medications following 1992 animal studies that suggested a cancer risk. The BGA recommends daily pyrrolizidinalkaloid intake not to exceed one milligram, as determined by recommended dosages on product labels. Since the 1980s, Weber & Weber has produced a patented butterbur root extract with undetectable concentrations of pyrrolizidinalkaloids, providing a product with no potential risks. Ironically, past studies have shown butterbur root to be a viable treatment for cancer in that it appears to stop the spread (metastasis) of some cancer cells.

Kava (*Piper methysticum*): A root native to the South Pacific, kava has been used for centuries as a calmative botanical. Its primary application is to relax the central nervous system and promote sleep. Recently, its ability to relax muscles has also emerged. A German study published in a 1995 issue of *Neuropharmacology* reported that the pyrone compounds found in kava have both pain killing and muscle relaxing properties. If your incontinence is due to muscle spasms, this herb may be of benefit to you.

Recommended Dosage: Take forty-five to seventy milligrams of kavalactones three times daily during a sciatica flare up. *Note:* Kava dosages depend on the kavalactone content of the kava supplement. Do not exceed recommended doses or combine kava with benzodiazepine drugs.

HERBS FOR INCONTINENCE CAUSED BY NERVE DYSFUNCTION

Ginkgo (*Ginkgo biloba*): The bilobalide compounds found in the *Ginkgo biloba* leaf can contribute to nerve regeneration, which may be of value in certain forms of incontinence that are due to poor nerve feed to bladder muscles. An Italian study published in a 1993 issue of *Planta Medica* found that the percentage of muscle cells receiving nerve impulses was greatly enhanced in test animals treated with bilobalide. The data suggests that ginkgo worked to boost the regeneration and protection of neurons, which resulted in a better nerve feed to adjacent muscles. Italian researchers also discovered that ginkgo extracts have the ability to relax smooth muscle.

Recommended Dosage: Take forty to eighty milligrams three times daily of a ginkgo supplement standardized to contain 24 percent ginkgo flavonglycosides.

HERBS FOR INCONTINENCE CAUSED BY RECURRING BLADDER INFECTIONS

Cranberry (*Vaccinium macrocarpon*): If recurring bladder infections are behind your incontinence, cranberry extracts can be of great value. Cranberry is considered a superior herb for the treatment and prevention of bladder infections. Compounds in cranberry have the ability to inhibit *E. coli* bacteria from sticking to the walls of the bladder. Cranberry also has astringent applications for the urinary tract and acts as a natural diuretic and urinary antiseptic agent.

Eighty-five percent of urinary tract infections are caused by *E. coli*, a bacterium that resides in the large intestine where it contributes to friendly flora action. When it makes its way into the urethra and the bladder, however, an infection can result. The remaining 15 percent of bladder infections are caused by other bacteria that also live in the bowel. Bacteria must cling to the walls of the bladder to cause an infection; free-floating bacteria in urine are washed away and do not cause inflammation. When bacteria colonize in the walls of the bladder, destructive enzymes are released that destroy the bladder lining. As a result, capillary bleeding occurs, which explains why finding blood in the urine is a common symptom of a bladder infection.

After experimenting with various theories, it was concluded that cranberry contains a natural substance that keeps these bacteria from adhering to the bladder wall so they are flushed out in the urine instead. This active anti-adherence ingredient is currently in the process of becoming a patented medicine. Clinical trials involving double-blind studies found that 70 percent of urinary tract infections in women could be prevented with cranberry supplementation.

Recommended Dosage: Cranberry capsules can be taken more efficiently in stronger concentrations than juice. If you prefer to take juice, make sure it is pure, 100 percent unsweetened cranberry juice. This type of juice may not be found in grocery stores; check your local health food store. Drink at least one quart of juice daily. If you take capsules, start with four capsules per day for the first three to five days, and then drop down to two capsules per day. Take the capsules with a large glass of pure water or cranberry juice.

Possible Side Effects: None are known to date.

Corn silk (*Zea mays*): Corn silk refers to the soft, hair-like growth that accompanies an ear of corn. Corn silk compounds, which include maizenic acid, can act as a diuretic. Used by the ancient Incas as a treatment for urogenital infections, corn silk was marketed by Parke-Davis in Europe in 1880.

Corn silk is considered part of a family of herbs that help soothe and heal the urinary system. Clinical studies in China and Japan have demonstrated the remarkable diuretic properties of corn silk. Corn silk directly reduces painful symptoms and swelling due to several inflammatory conditions, including bladder infections and the production of scant urine.

Recommended Dosage: Take corn silk in appropriate doses as directed. Any substance that acts as a diuretic may cause a potassium deficiency if used in excess, so use potassium supplementation. Possible Side Effects: Corn silk is considered a mild, nontoxic herb. No side effects have been reported.

Uva Ursi (*Arctostaphylos uva-ursi*): Uva ursi is one of the best researched diuretics and has excellent antiseptic and antibacterial actions due to its arbutin content, which is converted to hydroquinone in the body. Uva ursi has the ability to drain excess water from the cells, thereby promoting an antiseptic effect on the kidneys. It also reduces the acidity of the urine. The arbutin content of uva ursi is responsible for its diuretic action. In addition, when it is excreted from the kidneys, arbutin produces an antiseptic effect on the mucous membranes of the urinary tract. Research has found that uva ursi is effective against nephritis and kidney stones and possesses all-around tonic properties. Clinical studies have indicated that it actually works to prevent the recurrence of bladder infections.

Recommended Dosage: Take only as directed. Usual dosages are between 250 to 500 milligrams daily of capsulized, dried uva ursi with a 10 percent arbutin content.

Possible Side Effects: Do not take this herb if you are pregnant or nursing, and do not exceed recommended dosages.

Goldenseal (*Hydrastis canadensis*): Used by Native Americans for generations, goldenseal root is a favorite among herbalists for its anti-inflammatory effect and antibiotic-like actions. Laboratory tests have proven goldenseal's ability to protect against gram-positive and gram-negative bacteria. Tests have found that this berberine-containing herb can be more effective in treating some infections than standard antibiotics.

Recommended Dosage: Take 200 to 500 milligrams daily of a product with an 8 percent alkaloid content.

Possible Side Effects: Do not use goldenseal if you are pregnant or nursing. Prolonged or excessive use may kill bacterial flora and raise white blood count. Taking unusually high amounts of goldenseal can lower heartbeat and adversely affect the central nervous system.

Continual use can lower vitamin-B absorption. Goldenseal is not recommended for anyone with low blood sugar or hypertension.

Vitamin A: This vitamin is essential for healthy skin and proper function of the eyes. Vitamin A is also important for the immune system.
Recommended Dosage: Take 25,000 to 50,000 IU daily. Pregnant women should not exceed 25,000 IU daily.

Vitamin C: This vitamin is necessary for healthy tissue growth and maintenance. Vitamin C is an antioxidant and is well known for its role in strengthening the immune system.
Recommended Dosage: Take 500 milligrams three to five times daily.

Zinc: An important trace mineral, zinc aids the immune system and enzymatic activity related to cell growth and division.
Recommended Dosage: Take 30 milligrams daily.

Acidophilus: A bacteria found in yogurt, acidophilus helps restore a balanced bacterial environment in the intestinal tract.
Recommended Dosage: Use either liquid or capsules twice a day. Look for products with bifidobacteria, and check the expiration date.

HERBS FOR INCONTINENCE CAUSED BY PROSTATE ENLARGEMENT OR INFLAMMATION

Pygeum: Native to areas of Africa and Madagascar, this evergreen tree has traditionally been used to make a tea for genito-urinary disorders. Today, standardized extracts of pygeum are used for prostatic hyperplasia, enlarged prostate or BPH. The herb has also been used in people who have scant urine or who produce an excess amount of urine and find that they must urinate several times during the night.

The phytosterols contained in pygeum have anti-inflammatory properties that inhibit the formation of prostaglandins, which are responsible for the swelling in the prostate. One of these phytosterols, betasitosterol, has been shown to be helpful in cases of BPH. The pentacyclic triterpenoids of pygeum also work to block the enzymatic activity associated with inflammation and swelling in the prostate gland. Both actions help restore normal urination. *Recommended Dosage:* Use 50 to 100 milligrams twice daily of a product standardized to contain a 14 percent triterpene and beta-sitosterol content and a 0.5 percent n-docosanol content. *Possible Side Effects:* No toxicity has been reported with pygeum.

Saw Palmetto (*Serenoa repens*): The saw palmetto berry was used by ancient Mayans to treat disorders of the genito-urinary tract. Interestingly, today scientists are discovering that compounds in saw palmetto can prevent the conversion of testosterone to dihydrotestosterone, which helps to prevent the development of prostate disease. The ability of saw palmetto to treat prostate disease has been the subject of recent clinical studies. The results of these studies have been impressive and strongly suggest that saw palmetto may be a viable alternative to Proscar, a pharmaceutical drug used for treating an enlarged prostate gland. Saw palmetto may also be useful for women who suffer from hormonal imbalances by helping to normalize estrogen levels, which can also help to control certain kinds of incontinence. *Recommended Dosage:* Take 160 milligrams twice daily of a product with a standardized extract that contains 85–95 percent of fatty acids and sterols. *Possible Side Effects:* No toxicity has been reported.

Zinc: Zinc is necessary for optimal immune function. A deficiency of zinc has been related to increased occurrence of infections. *Recommended Dosage:* Take forty-five to sixty milligrams daily.

Flaxseed Oil: Flaxseed oil is a rich source of omega-3 fatty acids, which are necessary for normal cell structure. Omega-3 fatty acids also promote cardiovascular health. *Recommended Dosage:* Take one tablespoon daily.

HERBS FOR INCONTINENCE CAUSED BY KIDNEY STONES

Juniper (*Juniperus communis*): Known for its aromatic blue-green berries, juniper has been used in Europe to treat kidney disorders, urinary tract infections and prostate disease. It has blood-purifying and antiseptic properties that make it a natural treatment for disorders affecting the urinary system. Juniper acts directly on kidney function by increasing the rate of glomerulus filtration (blood purification) to stimulate urine flow.

Studies have found that juniper can help restore kidney tissue and normalize blood pressure after kidney disease. Juniper effectively expels uric acid from the body, which helps to prevent the development of kidney stones.

Recommended Dosage: Take as directed on product label.

Possible Side Effects: Long term or excessive use may cause kidney irritation or inhibit iron absorption. If pregnant, use juniper only with your physician's permission.

Couch grass (*Agropyron repens*): This herb is a natural diuretic that helps to control bladder infections. Couch grass can stimulate urine discharge. Extracts of couch grass have exhibited antibiotic effects on a variety of bacteria and molds, and some experts believe that couch grass can help to eliminate kidney stones, although more research is needed.

Recommended Dosage: Take as directed on product label.

Possible Side Effects: Take appropriate doses as recommended; an excess of couch grass could lead to potassium and other mineral deficiencies.

DIURETIC HERBS FOR CLEANSING THE URINARY TRACT

Parsley: Much more than a garnish, parsley supplies chlorophyll and helps to restore urinary tract health. The diuretic action of this herb is due to compounds called myristicin and apiole. Parsley is used in Britain and Germany to provide irrigation when treating kidney stones. Studies have shown that in comparison to citrus juices, parsley contains three times more vitamin C, gram per gram. The flavonoid content of parsley stimulates normal urination.

Recommended Dosage: Use as directed on product label.

Possible Side Effects: Pregnant women should not use excessive amounts of parsley.

Dandelion (*Taraxacum officinale*): Rich in potassium, dandelion works to detoxify the blood and is considered a powerful natural diuretic. Modern research has proven that dandelion can stimulate the elimination of uric acid from the body. One study indicates that dandelion has diuretic activity that compares to furosemide (Lasix), a prescription drug.
Recommended Dosage: Take 200 to 500 milligrams daily.
Possible Side Effects: None are known to date.

NATURAL COMPOUNDS THAT HELP INCREASE MUSCLE TONE

Malic acid: Malic acid participates in muscle cell metabolic processes that help muscles to use glucose properly.
Suggested Dosage: Take 300 milligrams three times daily with a magnesium supplement.

Magnesium: Magnesium works to support muscle cell function and has a synergistic action when combined with malic acid.
Suggested Dosage: Take 800 milligrams of magnesium daily. Use chelated products.

Grapeseed or Pinebark Extract: A powerful antioxidant and natural anti-inflammatory, this compound helps to inhibit the inflammatory response and scavenges for free radicals, which can cause muscle damage.
Suggested Dosage: Take as directed. You may want to start with a higher dose to saturate cells and then gradually lower the dose.

Coenzyme Q10: This enzyme helps to boost oxygen supplies to muscle tissue, as demonstrated in clinical studies on compromised heart muscle. Deficiencies of coenzyme Q10 have been found in the muscle mitochondria of people with muscular dystrophy.
Suggested Dosage: Use 100 milligrams daily in divided doses.

Glucosamine/Chondroitin: These compounds can help boost the production of collagen and exert a protective and regenerative effect on cartilage stores.

Suggested Dosage: Take 1,500 milligrams daily of glucosamine sulfate and 200 to 1,200 milligrams daily of chondroitin sulfate. (Look for supplements with manganese ascorbate.)

NADH: NADH helps to control pain and muscle spasms. *Suggested Dosage:* Take two to five milligrams once a day.

Ginkgo Biloba: This herb promotes better muscle cell oxygenation during periods of muscular stress.
Suggested Dosage: Take forty to eighty milligrams of a Ginkgo biloba supplement standardized to contain 24 percent ginkgo flavonglycosides three times daily.

Calcium/Magnesium: These nutrients are very important for proper muscle contraction and nerve function and should be taken as a supplement daily. A calcium deficiency can actually cause muscle cramping or other muscle problems. Magnesium increases the body's absorption of calcium. Taking a calcium/magnesium supplement at bedtime may help reduce pain and promote sleep.
Suggested Dosage: Take as directed on product label, using gluconate or citrate forms.

Carnitine: Carnitine is an amino acid that has been linked with muscle development and tone.
Suggested Dosage: Take as directed on product label, on an empty stomach and with a glass of fruit juice.

OTHER ALTERNATIVE THERAPIES FOR INCONTINENCE

The following therapies for incontinence can be practiced at home or administered by a qualified health care practitioner.

Yoga: Practicing yoga techniques, which are similar to Kegel exercises, is recommended. Contracting the pelvic floor and the vaginal sphincter and relaxing it several times can strengthen the set of muscles responsible for incontinence. (Aswini mudra is the name of this yoga exercise.)

Acupuncture: Several studies suggest that acupuncture can benefit some forms of incontinence. One clinical trial using a needle technique in the BL-33 sector (Zhongliao points) for four weeks among eight patients found that incontinence was controlled completely in three patients (38 percent) and partially controlled in three patients (38 percent). Researchers concluded that acupuncture could be a promising alternative to conventional therapies for urinary incontinence caused by detrusor hyperreflexia in patients with chronic spinal cord injuries. The beauty of acupuncture is that it is completely without side effects.

Hypnosis: In one study conducted by British researchers, fifty women with incontinence due to structural weakness received twelve sessions of hypnosis for one month: twenty-nine patients became entirely symptom free, fourteen improved, and seven remained unchanged. What this test suggested was that even though the incontinence was thought to be physical in origin, strong psychological factors existed that enabled hypnosis to work on actual body function and sensation. It was also discovered that women suffering from a detrusor instability incontinence were very good candidates for hypnosis.

Homeopathic Medicines: While research studies evaluating the benefit of homeopathic medicines for incontinence are scare, the following are traditional homeopathic medicines used to treat various kinds of incontinence:

- Arnica (leopard's bane) is used for involuntary urination after surgery.
- Belladonna (deadly nightshade) is recommended for people who suffer from dribbling urine.
- Ferrum phos (iron phosphate) and kreosotum (beechwood) are used for UI. Other homeopathic medicines for incontinence include aconite, apis mel and cantharis.

Hydrotherapy: Taking a sitz bath daily (especially with colder temperatures) has been helpful for some women with incontinence.

Tips for Managing Incontinence

- Avoid consuming anything that contains caffeine (such as coffee, tea, colas, chocolate and several over-the-counter and prescription drugs).
- Avoid carbonated drinks, alcohol, citrus juices, greasy and spicy foods and artificial sweeteners. All of these can actually irritate the bladder.
- Drink five to eight glasses of pure water throughout the day.
- Wear clothing that can be quickly changed even in public bathroom settings.
- Use pants and skirts with an elastic waist and shirts and blouses with snaps.
- Wear absorbent pads or briefs.
- Always empty your bladder before you leave the house, take a nap or retire for the evening.
- Go to the bathroom frequently before you feel the urge and when you urinate, empty your bladder thoroughly.
- Use an alarm clock or wristwatch alarm to remind you to go to the bathroom.
- Check with your doctor about the possibility of using a self-catheter. A self-catheter is a clear, straw-like device that is inserted into the opening of the urethra and assists you in emptying your bladder completely.
- Make sure your bathroom is very accessible and well lit, and keep the door open and the toilet seat up.
- If you have trouble getting on and off the toilet, try using an elevated padded toilet seat and installing hand rails to help you get on and off.
- Keep a bedpan, portable toilet or plastic urinal (for men) near your bed.

Tips for Controlling the Urge to Urinate

- Relax, and focus on slow, deep breathing. Concentrate on inhaling and exhaling and on your chest movements.
- Count backwards from 100, or sing all the lyrics to a particular song to distract your mind.

- When you are at home and the possibility of an accident poses less inconvenience, try to delay going to the bathroom for two minutes after you feel the urge; work up to delaying for five minutes.
- Practice walking slowly to the bathroom while you keep your mind distracted.
- Always empty your bladder immediately before going to sleep.

References

Avorn, J., et al. "Reduction of bacteriuria and pyuria after ingestion of cranberry juice." *JAMA* 271 (1994): 751–54.

Barron, J., et al. "Malate-aspartate shuttle, cytoplasmic NADH redox potential, and energetics in vascular smooth muscle." *J Mol Cell Cardiol* 30 (Aug. 1998): 1571–79.

Bauer, R., and H. Wagner. "Echinacea species as potential immunostimulatory drugs." *Econ Med Plant Res* 5 (1991): 253–321.

Berger, D., et al. "Influence of Petasites hybridus on dopamine-D2 and histamine-H1 receptors." *Pharm Acta Helv* 72 (Feb. 1998): 373–75.

Bickel, D., et al. "Identification and characterization of inhibitors of peptido-leukotriene-synthesis from Petasites hybridus," *Planta Med* 60 (Aug. 1994): 318–22.

Blaivas, Jerry. *Conquering Bladder and Prostate Problems: The Authoritative Guide for Men and Women.* New York, NY: Plenum, 1998.

Breitkreutz, R., et al. "Effect of carnitine on muscular glutamate uptake and intramuscular glutathione in malignant diseases." *Br J Cancer* 82 (Jan. 2000): 399–403.

Bruno, C., et al. "Regeneration of motor nerves in bilobalide-treated rats." *Planta Med* 59 (Aug. 1993): 302–7.

Carle, R. Pflanzliche Antiphlogistika und Spasmolytika, Zschr. Phytoth 9, 3 (1988): 67–76.

Chatelain, C., et al. "Comparison of once and twice daily dosage forms of Pygeum africanum extract in patients with benign prostatic hyperplasia: a randomized, double-blind study, with long-term open label extension." *Urology* 54 (Sept. 1999): 473–78.

Debrunner, B., and B. Meier. "Petasites hybridus: a tool for interdisciplinary research in phytotherapy." *Pharm Acta Helv* 72 (Feb. 1998): 359–62.

Freeman, R., et al. "Hypnotherapy for incontinence caused by the unstable detrusor." *Br Med J* (Clin Res Ed) 19 (Jun. 1982) (6332): 1831–34.

Gleitz, J., et al. "Kavain inhibits veratridine-activated voltage-dependent Na(+)-channels in synaptosomes prepared from rat cerebral cortex." *Neuropharmacology* 34 (Sept. 1995): 1133–38.

Goepel, M., et al. "Saw palmetto extracts potently and noncompetitively inhibit human alpha1-adrenoceptors in vitro." *Prostate* 15, 38 (3) (Feb. 1999): 208–15.

Honjo, H., et al. "Acupuncture for urinary incontinence in patients with chronic spinal cord injury." *Nippon Hinyokika Gakkai Zasshi* 89 (Jul. 1998): 665–69.

Jahodar, L., et al. "Antimicrobial effect of arbutin and an extract of the leaves of Arctostaphylos uva-ursi in vitro." *Cesk Farm* 34 (Jun. 1985): 174–78.

Kim, H. K., et al. "Inhibition of rat adjuvant-induced arthritis by ginkgetin, a biflavone from ginkgo biloba leaves." *Planta Med* 65 (Jun. 1999): 465–67.

King, Barbara, and Judy Harke. *Coping with Bowel and Bladder Problems*. San Diego: Singular Publishing Group, 1994.

Leung, A. *Encyclopedia of Common Natural Ingredients Used in Food, Drugs and Cosmetics*. New York: John Wiley and Sons, 1980.

Lin Y. L., et al. Four new sesquiterpenes from Petasites formosanus, National Research Institute of Chinese Medicine, Taipei 112, Taiwan, and Department of Chemistry, National Taiwan University, Taipei.

McKinney, D. "Saw palmetto for benign prostatic hyperplasia." *JAMA* 12; 281 (18) (May 1999): 1699.

Mowrey, Daniel. *The Scientific Validation of Herbal Medicine*. Connecticut: Keats Publishing, 1986.

Murray, Michael. *Encyclopedia of Nutritional Supplements*. Rocklin, CA: Prima Publishing, 1996.

Newman, D. "Entering the 21st century: moving incontinence treatment options to the forefront." *Ostomy Wound Manage* 45 (Dec. 1999): 5–6.

Nielsen, S., et al. "Effect of parsley (Petroselinum crispum) intake on urinary apigenin excretion, blood antioxidant enzymes and biomarkers for oxidative stress in human subjects." *Br J Nutr* 81 (Jun. 1999): 447–55.

Ode, P. *The Complete Medicinal Herbal*. New York: Dorling Kindersley, 1993.

Oei, H., et al. "Enuresis and encopresis as a reaction to food." *Ned Tijdschr Geneeskd* 133 (Aug. 5, 1989): 1555–57.

Prodromos, P., et al. "Cranberry juice in the treatment of urinary tract infections." *Southwestern Med* 47, 17 (1968).

Puglisi, L., et al. "Pharmacology of natural compounds. I. Smooth muscle relaxant activity induced by a Ginkgo biloba L. extract on guinea-pig trachea." *Pharmacol Res Commun* 20 (Jul. 1988): 573–89.

Rehman, J., et al. "Increased production of antigen-specific immunoglobulins G and M following in vivo treatment with the medicinal plants Echinacea angustifolia and Hydrastis canadensis." *Immunol Lett* 68 (2–3) (Jun. 1, 1999): 391–95.

Reid, G., et al. "Influence of three day antimicrobial therapy and lactobacillus vaginal suppositories on recurrence of urinary tract infections." *Clin Ther* 14 (1992): 11–16.

Rogers, J. "Pass the cranberry juice." *Nurs Times* 87 (Nov. 27–Dec. 3, 1991): 36–37.

Sabota, A. "Inhibition of bacterial adherence by cranberry juice: potential use for the treatment of urinary tract infections," *Journal of Urology* 131 (1984): 1013–16.

Sandroff, Ronni. "Urgent Matters: Incontinence is Treatable, if Only Women Would Talk about It." *American Health for Women* 18 (Oct. 1997): 28–30.

Tyler, V. E., L .R. Brady, and J. E. Robbers. *Pharmacognosy*. 7th ed. Philadelphia: Lead and Febiger, 1976.

Zafriri, D., et al. "Inhibitory activity of cranberry juice on adherence of type 1 and type P fimbriated Escherichia coli to eucaryotic cells." *Antimicrob Agents Chemother* 33 (Jan. 1989): 92–88.